The Fibroid

A complete guide to healing, managing and overcoming a common women's health challenge.

Donald V. Woodson

Disclaimer

The information in this publication is for general informational purposes only. While efforts have been made to ensure accuracy, the author and publisher make no warranties about the completeness or reliability of the content. Any actions taken based on this information are at your own risk.

The views expressed are those of the author and do not necessarily reflect those of any affiliated organizations. The author and publisher disclaim liability for any damages arising from the use of this publication.

This content is not intended as professional advice. For specific guidance, consult a qualified professional. By using this publication, you agree to indemnify the author and publisher from any claims or damages resulting from its use.

Table of Contents

Introduction

Uterine fibroids are a common yet often overlooked condition affecting millions of women. These non-cancerous growths in or around the uterus can range from being entirely unnoticed to causing significant health challenges. Despite their prevalence, fibroids are surrounded by misconceptions and unanswered questions. This book aims to demystify fibroids, offering a concise yet comprehensive guide to understanding their nature, symptoms, and treatment options. Through a blend of medical insights and personal stories, we provide a unique perspective on managing and living with fibroids. Whether you're newly diagnosed, a long-term warrior, or simply curious, this book is your essential companion in navigating the world of fibroids. Join us on this journey to clarity, empowerment, and better health.

Chapter 1

What are Fibroids

Fibroids, or uterine fibroids (leiomyomas), are benign tumors that form in or on the uterus. Composed of muscle and fibrous tissue, they can range in size. While many fibroids are asymptomatic, they can sometimes lead to heavy menstrual bleeding, pelvic discomfort, and pressure on nearby organs. Their growth is influenced by hormones such as estrogen and progesterone. Fibroids are especially common among women of childbearing age.

Fibroids are more prevalent between the ages of 30 and the onset of menopause. They commonly diminish after menopause. Between 20% and 80% of females developed fibroids by the age of 50, according to the Office on Women's Health (OWH).

Chapter 2

Types of Fibroid

1. Intramural Fibroids

Intramural fibroids are the foremost visit frame that start inside the muscle divider of the uterus. These fibroids may cause the uterus to appear broadened and may lead to side effects such as over the top month to month stream, pelvic distress, and weight. When intramural fibroids create adequately, they may misshape the ebb and flow of the uterus and affect ripeness.

2. Submucosal Fibroids

Submucosal fibroids begin specifically beneath the lining of the uterine depth (the endometrium). In spite of the fact that they are less predominant, they may create genuine indications, counting intemperate menstrual streams and extended periods. Submucosal fibroids may be too meddled with richness and pregnancy, expanding the chance of premature delivery and troubles amid pregnancy.

3. **Subserosal Fibroids**

Subserosal fibroids frame on the external surface of the uterus. As they grow, they may spread outward and apply weight on neighboring organs, such as the bladder and digestive system, coming about to side effects counting visit urination and clogging. Subserosal fibroids may too cause back and leg inconvenience in case they encroach on nerves.

4. **Pedunculated Fibroids**

Pedunculated fibroids are connected to the uterus by a slim stalk, either inside the uterine depression (submucosal) or on the exterior surface (subserosal). These fibroids may deliver strong discomfort if the stalk gets turned, cutting off the fibroid's blood supply (a condition known as torsion).

Less common
1.Cervical Fibroid

Cervical fibroids grow in the cervical region, which is the neck of the uterus. These fibroids are rare and can lead to several issues, including:

Pain During Intercourse: The presence of fibroids in the cervical area can make sexual intercourse uncomfortable or painful.

Bleeding: Cervical fibroids can cause abnormal bleeding, including spotting between periods or heavy menstrual bleeding.

Difficulties During Childbirth: Fibroids in the cervix can obstruct the birth canal, leading to complications during delivery.

2. Intraligamentous Fibroids

Intraligamentous fibroids develop in the ligaments that support the uterus, such as the broad ligament. These fibroids can cause:

Pelvic Pain: The growth of fibroids in the supportive ligaments can lead to significant pelvic discomfort.

Pressure on the Bladder or Bowel: As these fibroids grow, they can exert pressure on adjacent organs, leading to urinary and bowel symptoms, such as frequent urination or constipation.

3. Parasitic Fibroids

Parasitic fibroids are an uncommon type that occurs when a subserosal fibroid detaches from the uterus and reattaches to another organ. This detachment and reattachment allow the fibroid to receive its blood supply from the new location. Parasitic fibroids can cause:

Pain: The fibroid's new location can cause discomfort or pain, depending on which organ it attaches to.

Functional Disruption: Depending on the attachment site, these fibroids can interfere with the normal function of the affected organ, potentially leading to a range of symptoms.

Chapter 3

Causes of Fibroid

The specific etiology of fibroids is not entirely known, however numerous variables are considered to contribute to their development:

1. Hormones
Hormones have a crucial influence in the development of fibroids:
Estrogen and Progesterone: These hormones, which control the menstrual cycle, encourage the formation of the uterine lining. Fibroids possess more estrogen and progesterone receptors than normal uterine muscle cells, leading them to develop in response to these hormones. Fibroids tend to diminish after menopause owing to a drop in hormone levels.

2. Genetic Changes

Gene Mutations: Many fibroids have genetic changes that are distinct from those present in normal uterine muscle cells. These mutations may lead to the formation of fibroids.

3. Growth Factors

Insulin-like formation Factors: These molecules, which assist the body maintain tissues, may also impact the formation of fibroids.

4. Extracellular Matrix (ECM)

ECM Components: The ECM, which causes cells to stick together, is more plentiful in fibroids, making them fibrous. ECM retains growth substances and induces biological changes in cells.

Chapter 4

Risk Factors

Several risk factors enhance the possibility of acquiring fibroids:

1. Family History
Genetic Predisposition: Having a family member with fibroids doubles your risk. For example, if your mother or sister had fibroids, you are more likely to have them.

2. Race
Ethnicity: African-American women are more prone to acquire fibroids than women of other ethnic groupings. Additionally, they may get fibroids at earlier ages and have more severe symptoms.

3. Hormonal Factors
EarlyMenstruation:Starting menstruation at an early age raises the risk of fibroids.

Birth Control Use: Some kinds of birth control might impact hormone levels, possibly affecting fibroid formation.

4. Lifestyle and Health Factors
Obesity: Women who are overweight have an increased chance of acquiring fibroids. This may be related to elevated quantities of estrogen generated by fat cells.

Diet: A diet strong in red meat and poor in green vegetables, fruit, and dairy products may raise the incidence of fibroids.

Vitamin D Deficiency: Low levels of vitamin D are related to an increased incidence of fibroids.
Alcohol Consumption: Drinking alcohol, particularly beer, might raise the risk of fibroids.

Chapter 5

Symptoms of Fibroid

Fibroids may produce a variety of symptoms, some of which may be distinctive and greatly influence a woman's quality of life. Understanding these symptoms may aid in early diagnosis and efficient treatment.

1. Heavy Menstrual Bleeding
•Menorrhagia: Prolonged and heavy menstrual bleeding is a frequent sign of fibroids. Women may suffer periods that extend more than a week, necessitating several changes of sanitary protection.

2. Pelvic Pain and Pressure
•Chronic Pelvic Discomfort: Fibroids may produce a continual dull aching or severe pain in the pelvic area. The size and placement of the fibroids might contribute to a sense of fullness or pressure in the lower abdomen.

•Pain During Intercourse: Known as dyspareunia, fibroids, particularly cervical and submucosal kinds, may make sexual intercourse unpleasant.

3. Urinary and Bowel Symptoms
•Frequent Urination: Large fibroids may push on the bladder, resulting in an increased desire to pee.

•Problems Emptying the Bladder: This pressure may also create problems in entirely emptying the bladder.

•Constipation and Bloating: Fibroids pushing on the rectum may produce constipation, bloating, and a sense of incomplete bowel motions.

4. Lower Back and Leg Pain Sciatica-like Symptoms: Fibroids may push on nerves, producing pain that spreads down the back and legs, similar to sciatica.

5. Reproductive Issues
•Infertility: Fibroids may interfere with the implantation of an embryo or obstruct the fallopian tubes, making it difficult to conceive.

•Issues During Pregnancy: Fibroids may lead to an increased chance of miscarriage, premature delivery, and issues during labor, such as obstructed labor.

6. Abnormal Bleeding
•Intermenstrual Bleeding: Some women have spotting or bleeding between periods.

•Postmenopausal Bleeding: Fibroids may induce bleeding after menopause, which is not common and demands medical examination.

7. Anemia
•Iron-Deficiency Anemia: Heavy monthly flow may lead to anemia, marked by tiredness, weakness, and pale complexion.

8. Enlarged Abdomen
•Abdominal Distension: Large fibroids may produce visible swelling in the lower abdomen, commonly misinterpreted for weight gain or pregnancy.

9. Impact on Quality of Life
•Emotional and Psychological Stress: The persistent pain and discomfort associated with fibroids may lead to worry, sadness, and a considerable deterioration in quality of life.

Chapter 6

Effect of Fibroid in Pregnancy

1. Elevated Miscarriage Risk

- **Early Pregnancy Loss**: Fibroids, particularly submucosal ones that alter the uterine cavity, can disrupt embryo implantation and growth, leading to a higher risk of first-trimester miscarriages.

2. Preterm Labor and Birth

- **Premature Delivery**: The presence of fibroids can cause the uterus to overstretch, initiating early labor. Women with large or multiple fibroids face a greater risk of delivering prematurely, potentially leading to newborn complications.

3. Placental Issues

- **Placenta Previa**: Fibroids can impact the placenta's position, sometimes causing placenta previa, where the placenta covers the cervix, heightening the risk of bleeding during pregnancy and childbirth.
- **Placental Abruption**: Fibroids increase the likelihood of placental abruption, where the placenta detaches from the uterine wall prematurely, posing serious threats to both mother and baby.

4. Restricted Fetal Growth

- **Intrauterine Growth Restriction (IUGR)**: Fibroids can limit the space for fetal development, leading to IUGR, where the baby is smaller than expected for the gestational age, resulting in potential health issues.

5. Abnormal Fetal Positions

- **Malpresentation**: Fibroids can alter the uterine shape, causing the baby to settle in unusual positions like breech (feet or buttocks first) or transverse (sideways), complicating vaginal delivery and increasing the likelihood of a cesarean section.

6. Labor Challenges

- **Obstructed Labor**: Large fibroids near the cervix or lower uterus can block the birth canal, causing obstructed labor and requiring a cesarean delivery.
- **Inefficient Labor**: Fibroids can interfere with effective uterine contractions during labor, prolonging labor and increasing the need for medical interventions like oxytocin augmentation or a cesarean section.

7. Postpartum Hemorrhage

- **Excessive Bleeding**: Fibroids can elevate the risk of postpartum hemorrhage, a potentially life-threatening condition where the uterus doesn't contract properly after delivery, leading to significant bleeding.

8. Higher Cesarean Delivery Rate

- **Increased C-Section Likelihood**: Due to complications such as obstructed labor, abnormal fetal positions, and placenta previa, women with fibroids are more likely to need a cesarean delivery.

9. Complicated Postpartum Recovery

- **Prolonged Recovery**: The presence of fibroids can complicate postpartum recovery, resulting in extended bleeding, pain, and a slower return to normal activities.

10. Psychological Effects

- **Emotional Strain and Anxiety**: The potential pregnancy complications associated with fibroids can cause significant emotional stress and anxiety for expectant mothers, affecting their overall pregnancy experience and mental well-being.

Chapter 7

Effect of Fibroid on Fertility

Fibroids can greatly influence fertility, presenting various challenges for women attempting to conceive. Understanding these impacts is essential for addressing fertility issues and seeking appropriate treatment.

1. Distortion of the Uterine Cavity

- **Interference with Conception**: Submucosal fibroids, which extend into the uterine cavity, can distort its shape. This distortion can hinder embryo implantation, reducing the likelihood of successful conception.

2. Tubal Obstruction

- **Blockage of Fallopian Tubes**: Fibroids situated near the fallopian tubes can obstruct the passage of sperm to the egg or impede the movement of a fertilized egg to the uterus. This physical blockage can prevent natural conception.

3. Altered Blood Flow

- **Reduced Uterine Blood Flow**: Large fibroids can change the blood flow to the uterine lining, affecting the endometrium's ability to support embryo implantation and early development. This compromised blood flow can lead to difficulties in achieving and maintaining a pregnancy.

4. Hormonal Imbalance

- **Changes in the Hormonal Environment**: Fibroids can disrupt the hormonal balance within the uterus, affecting the endometrium's receptivity to an embryo. This imbalance can complicate efforts to conceive.

5. Increased Risk of Miscarriage

- **Early Pregnancy Loss**: Fibroids, particularly those that distort the uterine cavity or invade the endometrial lining, can increase the risk of miscarriage in early pregnancy. The altered environment can make it difficult for an embryo to thrive.

6. Challenges with Assisted Reproductive Technology (ART)

- **Complications with IVF**: Fibroids can impact the success rates of assisted reproductive technologies like in vitro fertilization (IVF). They can interfere with embryo placement in the uterus, reduce implantation rates, and increase the likelihood of complications during pregnancy.

7. Ovarian Impact

- **Effects on Egg Quality**: Although less common, fibroids can sometimes affect the ovaries, influencing egg quality and overall ovarian function. This can further challenge achieving pregnancy.

8. Emotional Toll

- **Psychological Stress**: The stress and anxiety related to fertility challenges caused by fibroids can impact overall reproductive health. The emotional burden can affect hormonal balance and general well-being, further complicating efforts to conceive

Chapter 8

Foods that may help Fibroid shrink

1. Green Leafy Vegetables

Packed with Nutrients: Vegetables like spinach, kale, and Swiss chard are rich in vitamins, minerals, and antioxidants. These components help balance hormones and reduce inflammation, potentially curbing fibroid growth.

2. Cruciferous Vegetables

Detox Champions: Broccoli, cauliflower, Brussels sprouts, and cabbage contain compounds that aid liver detoxification and hormone metabolism, helping to lower excess estrogen levels that can promote fibroid growth.

3. Fruits

Antioxidant Powerhouses: Berries, citrus fruits, apples, and grapes are loaded with antioxidants, vitamins, and fiber. These nutrients help reduce inflammation and support the body's detoxification processes, which may help shrink fibroids.

4. Whole Grains

High-Fiber Choices: Whole grains such as oats, quinoa, brown rice, and barley are rich in fiber. This helps regulate blood sugar levels and support healthy digestion, reducing the risk of hormonal imbalances that can lead to fibroid growth.

5. Flaxseeds

Hormonal Regulators: Flaxseeds are rich in lignans, which can help balance estrogen levels in the body. Incorporating ground flaxseeds into your diet may support hormone regulation and potentially reduce fibroid growth.

6. Nuts and Seeds

Healthy Fats and Protein Sources: Almonds, walnuts, chia seeds, and pumpkin seeds provide healthy fats and protein. They also offer fiber and essential nutrients that support hormonal balance and overall health.

7. Fish

Rich in Omega-3s: Fatty fish like salmon, mackerel, sardines, and trout are high in omega-3 fatty acids, which have anti-inflammatory properties. Reducing inflammation can help manage fibroid symptoms and potentially shrink their size.

8. Legumes

Plant-Based Protein: Beans, lentils, chickpeas, and peas are excellent sources of plant-based protein and fiber. They support healthy digestion and help balance blood sugar levels, contributing to hormonal equilibrium.

9. Herbal Teas

Supportive Beverages: Teas like green tea, chamomile, and dandelion root are rich in antioxidants and anti-inflammatory compounds. These teas can support liver function and overall health, potentially aiding in fibroid reduction.

10. Water

Essential Hydration: Staying hydrated is vital for overall health. Drinking plenty of water helps flush toxins from the body, supports liver function, and maintains healthy tissue, including the uterus.

Additional Tips for Managing Fibroids

Limit Red Meat and Processed Foods: These can contribute to inflammation and hormonal imbalances.

Avoid Excessive Alcohol and Caffeine: These can affect hormone levels and exacerbate fibroid symptoms.

Exercise Regularly: Physical activity helps regulate hormones and reduce inflammation.

Manage Stress: Chronic stress can impact hormone balance, so practicing stress-reducing techniques like yoga, meditation, or deep breathing exercises can be beneficial.

Chapter 9

Best Treatment Options for Fibroids

Uterine leiomyomas, or fibroids, are benign tumors that may affect fertility, pelvic discomfort, and excessive monthly flow, among other symptoms. Although not all fibroids need therapy, there are a number of helpful choices for those dealing with severe symptoms. A patient's reproductive objectives, general health, and the size, number, and location of their fibroids all play a role in determining the optimal course of therapy for these benign tumors.

1. medication-based hormonal therapy, which may reduce estrogen and progesterone levels and decrease fibroids. One such medication is

gonadotropin-releasing hormone (GnRH) agonists. Prior to surgery, these therapies are often used to decrease the size of fibroid.

Hormonal contraceptives, such as oral contraceptives and intrauterine devices (IUDs), may alleviate the severe bleeding and discomfort caused by fibroids.

To alleviate symptoms such as pain and excessive bleeding, non-hormonal medications may be used, such as tranexamic acid and nonsteroidal anti-inflammatory medicines (NSAIDs).

2. Procedures with Minimal Invasion

The goal of the uterine fibroids embolization (UFE) technique is to reduce the size of the tumors by cutting off their blood supply. For women who would prefer not to have surgery but yet wish to keep their uterus, this is a viable alternative.

MRI-Guided Focused Ultrasound Surgery (FUS): This non-invasive method employs high-intensity ultrasound waves to heat and kill fibroid tissue.

3. Surgical Options

Myomectomy: This procedure includes the excision of fibroids while keeping the uterus. It's a wonderful alternative for ladies who seek to retain their fertility.

Hysterectomy: This final surgical surgery includes the removal of the uterus and is regarded as the most effective therapy for fibroids. It is indicated for women who have finished their families or do not wish further babies.

4. Lifestyle and Dietary Changes

Diet and Exercise: Maintaining a healthy weight via diet and exercise may help control fibroid symptoms. Some studies show that a diet rich in fruits, vegetables, and low in red meat may minimize the chance of getting fibroids.

Stress Management: Practices such as yoga, meditation, and acupuncture might help control the stress that may increase fibroid symptoms.

5. Natural and Alternative Treatments

Herbal Remedies: Some women experience relief from fibroid symptoms utilizing herbal medicines such as green tea extract, curcumin, and vitex (chasteberry). Always speak with a healthcare practitioner before commencing any herbal remedies.

Acupuncture: This traditional Chinese medical practice may help reduce pain and other symptoms linked with fibroids.

Chapter 10

Diagnosis of Fibroid

Medical history, physical examination, and imaging procedures are all part of the diagnostic process for fibroids, which are also called uterine leiomyomas. In order to successfully manage symptoms and choose the right therapy, an accurate diagnosis is crucial. A brief outline of the steps used to detect fibroids is as follows:

1.   Patient Background and Examination

Medical Background: A thorough medical history is required to diagnose fibroids. During this interview, the doctor will inquire about the patient's menstrual cycle, any symptoms (such as heavy bleeding, pelvic discomfort, or problems with fertility or pregnancy), and any other relevant medical history.

Medical Checkup: In order to detect any uterine anomalies, a pelvic examination is carried out. A doctor may detect fibroids by feeling the uterus, which can reveal its size and form.

Section 2: Imaging Methods

•Ultrasound: Pelvic ultrasound is the most frequent imaging tool used to identify fibroids. It employs sound waves to make pictures of the uterus and may be conducted transabdominally (through the belly) or transvaginally (through the vagina). Ultrasound helps assess the size, quantity, and location of fibroids.

•MRI (Magnetic Resonance Imaging): MRI offers a more detailed view of fibroids and is especially valuable for mapping the precise size and position of each fibroid. It is typically utilized while contemplating surgical alternatives or when ultrasonography findings are equivocal.

•Hysterosonography (Sonohysterography): This unique form of ultrasound includes injecting saline into the uterus to enlarge the uterine cavity, enabling a better picture of submucosal fibroids and other uterine abnormalities.

3. Additional Diagnostic Procedures

•Hysteroscopy: In this operation, a tiny, illuminated telescope (hysteroscope) is passed through the cervix into the uterus, enabling the doctor to observe the interior of the uterine cavity directly. This is especially beneficial for identifying submucosal fibroids.

•Laparoscopy: This minimally invasive surgical treatment includes inserting a laparoscope (a tiny camera) via a small incision in the belly. It enables the doctor to observe the exterior of the uterus and other pelvic organs and may be used to identify and occasionally cure fibroids.

•Endometrial Biopsy: Although not commonly used to identify fibroids, an endometrial biopsy may be done to rule out other disorders, such as endometrial hyperplasia or malignancy, especially in women with abnormal uterine bleeding.

4. Blood Tests

•Complete Blood Count (CBC): A CBC may be requested to screen for anemia owing to excessive monthly flow, a frequent sign of fibroids.

•Hormonal Tests: These tests may help analyze hormone levels and rule out other ailments that may produce similar symptoms, such as thyroid issues.

Chapter 11

Fibroid And Mental Health

1. Persistent agony and Discomfort

•Persistent Pain: Fibroids cause discomfort and agony all the time, which might make you anxious and stressed all the time. Physical and emotional tolls of living with chronic pain may wear people down to the point that they no longer enjoy life.

•Problems sleeping due to pain or excessive bleeding may make it hard to fall or stay asleep, which in turn can make you feel tired and irritable, all of which can worsen mental health problems.

2. Effect on Everyday Life

•Restrictions on Physical Activity: Fibroids' physical symptoms might make it difficult to do things you normally would, which can make you feel frustrated and powerless. Isolation and despair may set in as a result of this constraint.

•Profession and Personal Life: Dealing with discomfort, frequent doctor's visits, and excessive bleeding may make it difficult to focus on work and social activities, which in turn can lead to feelings of worry and stress.

3. Issues Regarding Procreation

• Infertility: The emotional toll on women dealing with fibroids-related infertility may be substantial. Depression and anxiety are common outcomes of the stress and lethargic lifestyle that accompanies infertility.

•Pregnancy Complications: Concerns about the influence of fibroids on pregnancy and delivery may cause substantial concern and mental pain.

4. Body Image and Self-Esteem

•Physical Changes: The presence of fibroids may lead to obvious changes in body form and size, altering body image and self-esteem. Women may feel self-conscious or humiliated, which may significantly affect their mental health.

•Sexual Health: Pain during intercourse and worries about body image may disrupt sexual relationships and intimacy, leading to mental anguish and a decline in general well-being.

5. Hormonal Influence

• Mood Swings: Hormonal imbalances linked with fibroids might lead to mood swings and emotional instability. Fluctuations in estrogen and progesterone levels may influence neurotransmitter activity, impacting mood and mental health.

Chapter 12

Lifestyle and Dietary Management

Lifestyle Modifications

1. Regular Physical exercise -Exercise: Engaging in regular physical exercise may help maintain a healthy weight and lower the levels of certain hormones that lead to fibroid development. Most days of the week, try to get at least thirty minutes of moderate exercise—walking, swimming, or cycling.

•Yoga and Stretching: Incorporating yoga and stretching activities may help ease pelvic discomfort and reduce stress, which can worsen fibroid symptoms.

2. Stress Management

•Mindfulness and Meditation: Practices such as mindfulness meditation, deep breathing exercises, and progressive muscle relaxation may help regulate stress levels and enhance general well-being.

•Adequate Sleep: Ensuring adequate and quality sleep is vital for hormone control and general wellness. Aim for seven to nine hours of sleep each night.

3. Avoiding Environmental Toxins

•Reduce Exposure: Limiting exposure to environmental pollutants, including as pesticides, plastics, and certain chemicals, might help lessen the risk of hormonal abnormalities that lead to fibroid development. Choose organic vegetables wherever feasible and avoid using plastic containers for food storage.

4. Regular Medical Check-ups

•Monitor Health: Regular visits to a healthcare practitioner may help monitor the development of fibroids and manage symptoms efficiently. Early identification and care are crucial to avoiding problems.

Dietary Modifications

1. Increase Intake of Fruits and Vegetables

•Nutrient-Rich Choices: Consuming a variety of fruits and vegetables delivers critical vitamins, minerals, and antioxidants that promote general health and hormonal balance. Leafy greens, berries, citrus fruits, and cruciferous veggies like broccoli and cauliflower are especially helpful.

•Anti-Inflammatory Properties: Foods rich in antioxidants and anti-inflammatory chemicals may help decrease inflammation and perhaps limit fibroid development.

2. Choose Whole Grains

•Fiber-Rich Foods: Whole grains such as oats, quinoa, brown rice, and barley are rich in fiber, which helps control blood sugar levels and promote good digestion. Balanced blood sugar levels may lower the danger of hormonal abnormalities that lead to fibroid development.

3. Incorporate Healthy Fats

•Omega-3 Fatty Acids: Fatty fish like salmon, mackerel, sardines, and trout are rich in omega-3 fatty acids, which have anti-inflammatory qualities. Incorporating them into your diet may help control fibroid symptoms.

•Nuts and Seeds: Almonds, walnuts, chia seeds, and flaxseeds give healthful fats and vital nutrients that maintain hormonal balance.

4. Limit Red Meat and Processed Foods

•Reduce Consumption: Reducing the consumption of red meat and processed foods may help lessen the chance of developing fibroids. These meals are generally heavy in harmful fats and chemicals that may trigger inflammation and hormone abnormalities.

5. Stay Hydrated

•Water Intake: Drinking sufficient water is crucial for general health and helps the body clear pollutants. Staying well-hydrated helps liver function and maintains healthy tissues, including the uterus.

6. Herbal Supplements

•Natural Remedies: Some women receive relief from fibroid symptoms utilizing herbal supplements such as green tea extract, curcumin, and vitex (chasteberry). Always contact a healthcare physician before beginning any herbal remedies to confirm they are safe and suited for your situation.